# Christian Healthy Living

I0410497

Essential Information About Having A Positive Mental Attitude, Healthier Eating Habits, Being More Active, And More

Daphene Baines, M.A.

# Christian Healthy Living

Visit the author's website at
Gettinginshapeafter40.com

Disclaimer

Although every attempt has been made to produce the most accurate and trustworthy information possible, Daphene Baines does not accept liability for any actions taken as a result of reading this publication. This publication is not intended as nutritional counseling.

# Check Out My Related Book

**THE DANIEL FAST DIET: A Guide on How Christians can Lose Weight and Gain Spiritual Strength With the Daniel Fast[1]**

**See all of the books my husband and I have published at**

**www.RobertBaines.org**

# Dedication and Acknowledgements

This book is first and foremost dedicated to my heavenly Father. He has given me the desire and the ability to write this book. I thank Him for allowing me to be a part of His wonderful family. He is such a great father. I am thankful for my Savior and Lord, Jesus Christ. It is because of my belief in His great sacrifice that I have the right to eternal life. I am also grateful for the precious gift of the Holy Spirit who is my comforter. Wow, I serve an awesome Trinity.

I thank God for allowing me to have a team of people who love and support me. I am thankful for all the clients of the YMCA of Greater Cincinnati, the Center for the Closing the Health Gap, my Southern Baptist Church family, and those I privately trained. You all have been very helpful in my growth as an instructor and writer. Thank you for your questions, attending the teachings, and practicing the various Christian Healthy living principles.

Words cannot express the appreciation and gratitude that I have for my friends and family. Let me start out with my friend, Pamela Crumbly. This young lady is so encouraging and is always sharing my story with others. My story is that I have lost over 140 pounds and kept it off for years. Thanks P.C., love you. I have to thank my girl, Alma Gatewood. Alma, you have been there for me for over 35 years. You are one of my closest friends. I also want to thank Lady Regina Lynch. Your friendship is very dear and special to me. Please continue to be YOU.

Now, to my one and only family. To my mom and sister, who went to heaven and left me here to take care of my two older brothers. Thank you so very much – smile. Melvin and Silvester Tucker, I hope this book will help you and your families become healthier. My daughters, Daphene L. and Desiraye L. Davis are the most beautiful young ladies I know. Please allow God to minister to you and your families through this book. Desiraye, I thank you for marrying a good man, Jared Davis, and having two awesome children, Jared Ashton Davis, Jr. (JJ) and LilyGrace (Lily).

I need to write another book about my wonderful, handsome, loving husband, Dr. Robert E. Baines, Jr. I have so much to thank you for. You are a GREAT man. I am getting all teary eyed just thinking about how you are such a great priest, protector, and provider. Thank you for encouraging me to write this book. You are an awesome role model.

# TABLE OF CONTENTS

# Introduction

Question – which of the following is most important to you? Would you like to have energy, look good, live a long and enjoyable life, and be around for family, friends, church, and community for years to come? Or would you like to avoid unnecessary sickness, pain, and being embarrassed about your looks or fitness level? I hope that all of the above is important to you.

You know that God wants you to be a wise steward of the body that He has placed in your trust, right? You know that you need to eat a healthy diet. You know that you need to exercise. But did you know that it really starts with a positive mental attitude? And did you know that the older we get, the more likely we are to have to deal with changes in our hormones and sicknesses?

The **purpose** of this book is to provide you with quality and helpful information on how to live a healthy lifestyle. You should live each day like it is the most important day of your life. The decisions and actions you take will impact the rest of your life. Take your health seriously. Healthy living allows a person to perform daily activities, carry out leisure events, and respond to emergency situations with comfort and ease. Healthy living calls for a positive mental attitude, healthy eating, and physical activity.

## This is Personal

I am thankful that God helped me become conscious of my health and make some changes, while I still had time. I weighed 280 pounds after the birth of my baby and was up to 289 pounds, by my six week check-up. But with God's help, diet, exercise, determination, and a strong support system, I have kept over 140 pounds off. I have ran 5Ks, 10ks, 15ks, and my last run was a half marathon (i.e., 13.1 miles at 49 years old).

One of the primary reasons for me writing this book is to encourage other people, especially my two beautiful daughters, to set health goals and go for them. It will **not** be easy, but it is possible. Your journey and reason to get healthy may be different from mine. Whatever reason you have, make the decision, and take a step towards getting healthy.

# Problem Solving

As a trained wellness consultant and a certified life coach, I recommend everyone learn how to problem solve. Problem solving will move you from a seated position of being a victim to being a forward marching person of victory.

The first step in problem solving is to "recognize the problem." Denial of the issue does not solve the problem, it only delays the solving of the issue. On the Tom Joyner Morning Show (yes, I love this show), they regularly talk about "Deniabetes (i.e., denying diabetes)." It is important to define the problem, so that your focus is on the problem, not just the symptoms.

The second step is to "review the options." Look at the available options for handling the problem. For example, a person with diabetes may do research on the computer, go to the doctor, or just ignore the symptoms.

The third step is to "choose the best option." Continuing with the problem above, the best option may be going to the doctor.

The fourth step is "implementation." You must implement or do what you chose to do. In addition to just making the appointment, go to the appointment.

The fifth step is "evaluate and adjust as needed." Staying with our example, make sure you understand what the doctor told you, that you are following the instructions, and that the treatment is working. If you don't understand, adjust or solve that problem. If you are not following the instruction, adjust or solve that problem. If the treatment is not working, adjust or explore alternatives and go from there.

Remember, problem solving eliminates victims and creates victorious people. As you read through this book, be a victorious problem solver.

## Five Stages of Change

When going through change, we may experience the following emotions: fear, depression, anger, elation, excitement, and joy. The fitness community uses the five stages of change or the Transtheoretical Model, when helping people deal with change. This idea was introduced by Prochaska and DiClemente, in 1983 and updated by Prochaska, DiClemente, and Norcross, in 1992. As you read the five stages of change below, ask, "What stage of change are you in"?

1. Pre-contemplation. Here, you are not interested in changing, but you are bothered by something.

2. Contemplation. Here, you explore the possible benefits of changing.

3. Preparation. Here, you gather tools and support.

4. Action. Here, you take the steps necessary to change your life.

5. Maintenance. Here, you are able to maintain the change.

## How This Book is Organized

This book has four main sections. Section one looks at positive mental attitude. Section two is about healthy eating. Section three focuses on being more active. Section four deals with hormones and common sicknesses.

As we get started, remember this information is written to inspire you to make small changes towards a healthier you. "Rome was not built in a day." Read this book and decide what small change you will begin with, and add on, in the days and weeks that follow.

# Positive Mental Attitude

Let this mind be in you, which was also in Christ Jesus

- Philippians 2:5 (KJV)

"Health is not a condition of matter, but of the mind"

- Mary Baker

From the introductory material, let's focus on "positive mental attitude." In this chapter, we will discuss the following subjects:

- Your "why" statement
- Positive thinking
- Mediation
- Aromatherapy
- Yoga
- Sleep
- Happy foods

## Your "Why" Statement

Let's talk about why you want to do the challenging work of staying positive, as you work on your eating and activity level. Your motivation for doing this work needs to be clear to you.

A question to ask is, "Why should I want to change?" or "Why should I want to work on a healthier life style"? When your "why" is big enough, you will find your "how." Many are not successful with their plans, because they don't know "why" they started the plans or their "why" is not big enough.

As Christians, we should remember that I Corinthians 6:19-20 teaches us that "our" bodies actually belong to God, since He brought them with a price. Therefore, we should take care of our bodies, as items place in our trust for God's glory (see I Cor. 10:31). Please refer to my article, Temple of God: 6 Life Changing Comparisons About Your Body and God's Dwelling Place.[2]

How we take care of our health, in obedience to God's word, is a witness to the world. It is inconsistent to say I surrender all to the Lord and then eat a terrible diet and engage in very little activity (see Acts 1:8; I Cor. 10:31). Furthermore, taking care of your health will give you more energy to do what God is calling you to do. Which includes good works and enjoying abundant living (see Eph. 2:10; Jn. 10:10).

Other "whys" may include the following:

- I want to see my children (grandchildren) do well in life.
- I want to be able to travel and walk around comfortably, when I get to my destinations.
- I want to be able to serve in my church and community, after I retire.

**Motivation.** Motivation plays a pivotal role in having a positive mental attitude. Motivation simply means something that causes a person to act. Motivation may be called other words such as inspiration, incentive, drive, and enthusiasm.[3]

There are two kinds of motivation - extrinsic and intrinsic. Extrinsic motivation is the inspiration that comes from an external source, outside of you. It is something like when your health insurance gives you rewards for exercising and eating right. You find yourself getting involved with different plans for exercising and eating correctly, so you can win the rewards the insurance company has offered.

On the other hand, intrinsic motivation comes from within you. It is more like deciding to lose ten pounds, by next year, so you will feel better. Shape.com urges the use of intrinsic motivation to achieve long-term success (e.g., eating well and exercising makes them feel good). This can be done by setting some short-term and achievable goals, tracking your progress, and celebrating your success.

## Positive Thinking

It is important to remember that as a person think, so are they (see Pro. 23:7). If you **think** you cannot do something, you will not. But positive thinking can help you achieve your goals, and enjoy a better quality of life.

**Benefits.** The following are a few benefits of practicing positive thinking, even when things go wrong in your life:

- Mental and emotional refreshment
- Less stress
- Stay motivated
- Manage and enjoy your time in a better way
- Regulate blood pressure
- Eliminate emotional eating

- Improve your personal relationships.

**Tips.** Here are five simple tips to improving your positive thinking:

*1.   Try to see the positive side.* Stop worrying about things that you cannot control, and focus on things you can control. A positive thinker is able to recognize the true factors that led to an event and deal with them. Yes, give yourself time to grieve a failure, but try not to linger.

*2. Have a plan B.* "If at first you don't succeed, try, try, try again" is still true. Take time to relax and reflect on your actions. Consider other ways to succeed.

*3. Be cautious but not pessimistic.* Ask yourself are you being overly cautious, which can lead to pessimism and not trusting your own judgment.  Try not to let past failures prevent you from moving forward.

*4. Surround yourself with positive people.* It is true that staying positive is hard, especially when everyone around you is negative. So hang out with some positive people.

*5. Be Realistic.* Being positive is all about dealing with life's challenges in a positive way. It is NOT about ignoring danger signs.

**Affirmations.** Affirmations are a great tool to reinforce your positive thinking and open up to new possibilities. Essentially, they are short phrases that help you focus on your wants and needs and make them more specific. Instead of focusing on what is missing from your life, affirmations help you find ways to get what you want, by enforcing your will power and positive thinking. Affirmations work best when they are short, precise, and positive. In order to come up with the right affirmation for you, start by visualizing how great your life will be, once you achieve your goals. You may think of how you will be able to enjoy a day in the park with your children. Fitting into your little black dress and going to a play may be another visualization. Imagine being retired from your job without major illness may be something positive you want to think on.

Here are some examples of affirmations:[4]:

- I am most confident when I take care of myself.
- I am achieving my weight loss goals.

- I will succeed at reducing my weight.
- I choose to make positive healthy choices for myself.
- I can achieve and maintain my weight loss.
- I deserve to look my best.
- I am committed to healthy behavior and maintaining my beautiful body.
- I choose to exercise regularly.

**Questions.** Lifepossibilities.com is a great resource to find questions about life that will help you with a positive mental attitude. On their website is a list of 50 questions[5] that are helpful for reflection and meditation. The following are 10 questions that I like:

1. What's your passion?

2. What would you do in life, if you did not need to work for money?

3. Where do you want to be in 5, 10, 20, or 40 years?

4. Who are the three most important people in your life?

5. What is your biggest dream?

6. What are the three things in your life that you would like to change?

7. What are you grateful for?

8. Are you making the same mistakes over and over again?

9. When was the last time you helped someone?

10. What stops you from making the first step towards your dream?

**How Do I Keep The Pep In My Step?** Once you have gotten that spark, it is important to work on keeping it. The American Psychological Association offers a few ideas for doing this:

- Let yourself feel strong emotions. Then, learn how to manage what you do when you feel them.
- Do not avoid your problems. Learn how to meet the demands of daily living. You should also learn how to take a break and rest. Resting helps recharge your batteries.
- Spend time with loved ones. They can be great for support and

encouragement. At the same time, you must also take care of yourself.

- Give yourself a pat on the back every now and then. This is very important. If you do not tell yourself "good job," who will?

## Meditation

We are pulled in so many directions and have so much information to process on a daily basis that we often feel overwhelmed and uneasy. Meditation can be defined in many ways, but for me, it is returning to myself – coming back to my center and feeling at home there. The following are some benefits of meditation:

- It can help you stop harmful behaviors like smoking and overeating.
- It can lower your cholesterol levels and blood pressure.
- It can build self–confidence and help you get rid of phobias.
- It can increase your creativity and productivity.

In his book, Meditation Techniques, William Stanley says that meditation also does the following:

- Improved sleep and digestion
- Increase energy and aids weight loss
- Increased resilience
- Help relieve stress

Stanley says, "the consistent daily practice promotes the development of stability, inner calmness, and non-reactivity of the mind. In turn, this allows us to face and embrace even the unpleasant or painful aspects of daily life."

**Techniques.** If mediation is this beneficial, what is an effective way to meditate? William Stanley gives nine anxiety reducing mediation techniques. Let's look at three of these techniques.

1. Deep breathing. Make sure you sit in a comfortable position. Do some diaphragmatic breathing. That is, take a deep breath in through your nose letting your belly rise and fill with air. Hold. Exhale slowly through your nose (I recommend you exhale through your mouth). Hold. Repeat three times.

2. Body scan. This is when you focus your attention on different parts of your body. Stanley said this can be combined with deep breathing.

3. Daily activities. This technique is when you focus your attention on your everyday activities. This technique requires you to give your full attention to one thing at a time.  Please refer to William Stanley's book on meditation for more details about these and six other techniques.[6]

In the 2009 Humana.com newsletter, Maria Whitley wrote in her article, "Relax and Restore in Minutes a Day,"[7] about the following five tips for everyday relaxation and rejuvenation:

1. Sing in the shower. Singing reduces stress levels and elevates your mood.

2. Honor your life. People who practice gratitude can handle the negative effects of stress with greater ease.

3. Inner light. Let it shine, by taking a few minutes to breathe (see diaphragmatic breathing above).

4. Energize through movement. Stretch your body, before you get out of bed. Take

a moment to lie still. Notice how your body feels today, in the moment. Stretch after you stand up.

5. Nurture your body. By massaging your feet and hands with your favorite aroma and/or lotion in the morning or at night, you will increase blood flow into the area and relieve stress.

## Aromatherapy

Here is a quick word regarding aromatherapy and how it can be useful in meditation. According to Webmd.com Aromatherapy, or essential oils therapy, is using a plant's aroma-producing oils (essential oils) to treat disease.[8] Essential oils are taken from a plant's flowers, leaves, stalks, bark, rind, or roots. The oils are mixed with another substance (such as oil, alcohol, or lotion) and then put on the skin, sprayed in the air, or inhaled. You can also massage the oils into the skin or pour them into bath water. Aromatherapy as used today, originated in Europe and has been practiced there since the early 1900's.

Practitioners of aromatherapy believe that fragrances in the oils stimulate nerves in the nose. Those nerves send impulses to the part of the brain that controls memory and emotion. Depending on the type of oil, the result on the body may be calming or stimulating.

I believe that aromatherapy can aid a person who is practicing meditation. First, you need to discover what type of oil to use. A person can take a tour of a local aromatherapy or fragrance shop to discover the different types of fragrances. Getting a massage and asking about the different oils used can also be helpful. Reading the book Essential Oils for Beginners may be helpful.[9] This book does a great job describing the different oils and their benefits. Once the fragrance has been selected, a person can then take a meditative bath (i.e., warm water, soft music, sprinkle bath salt in the water, light a candle, put in two drops of your favorite oil, and turn off your phone) and begin to unwind. As you unwind, practice your breathing and mindfulness exercises.

## Yoga

Try yoga as a great tool with mediation. Yoga is known as a great de-stressor. Most gyms offer yoga classes, focusing mainly on the physical benefits that it offers, including increasing flexibility, toning of muscles, and lubricating the joints, ligaments, and tendons. Yoga has a hidden benefit of restoration. Yoga restores your spirit and reconnects you with your breath. Yoga means "to yoke," and it is this union of breath and body that renews you and brings harmony and peace of mind.

Yoga is beneficial for all body types and ages. You do not have to be flexible to do yoga, you just need to find the right class. The benefits are a more healthy and less stressful you.

## Sleep

Sleep is vital to having a positive mental attitude. Lack of sleep, according to WebMD.com, can have the following effects:[10]

- Cause accidents and increases risk of death
- Impair thinking, judgment, and memory
- Kills the sex drive
- Ages a person
- Makes a person gain weight

- Influences depression

**Benefits of Sleep.** According to Body and Soul, here are some reasons to get more sleep:[11]

1. You keep your figure and appear to be more attractive.

2. You can concentrate better, remember more clearly, and make better decisions.

3. You will be in a better mood.

4. You will be less likely to be ill.

5. You will live longer.

5. You will have better sex.

**Proper Amount of Sleep.** According to the National Sleep Foundation, one out of every three Americans sleeps six hours or less a night during the work week. The average American gets about seven hours of sleep a night, which is at the low end of the seven to nine hours experts say adults need. Infants need 18 hours; children need 10 to 12 hours; teens need 10 hours. The CDC says sleep deprivation is costing America $63 billion a year in lost productivity.

**Sleep Disorders.** From infants to adults, sleep disorders can be found. Some of these disorders require medical intervention. Others can be solved with milder remedies. Below are three common sleep problems and quick ways to treat them.

- Snoring. WebMD says to try changing your sleep position, losing weight, opening your nasal passage, get a new pillow, and drink water before you go to sleep.[12]
- Nightmares. Try to relax before going to bed, and do not watch scary movies or tell scary stories before bed.
- Sleep Apnea. Losing weight and following your doctor's orders will help.
- Teeth Grinding. Visit your dentist and get fitted for a guard. Over the counter guards are known to cause jaw pain.

Sleep is very important in having a positive mental attitude. Being tired will make a person irritated and agitated. Try to work on getting your proper sleep.

# Happy Foods

Happy foods are foods that help a person to feel more content. In the December 2014 Today Magazine, Rebecca Ungarino stated in her article, "5 Foods That May Make You Feel Happier Now — and Even Better Later" that some foods taste so good while we are eating them but can leave us feeling blah, bloated, and feeling guilty, moments after we have brushed away the crumbs. But other foods are scientifically shown to lift our spirits. She gives five foods that are helpful in lifting our spirits.[13]

1. Walnuts in their raw form, no sodium. Walnuts are a low-carb snack. An ounce of walnuts has 4 grams of protein (which fills you up and helps keep blood sugar levels steady) and 2 grams of fiber (also helps fill you up). They're also a good source of magnesium, antioxidants, and they are low in carbohydrates. Suggested serving: 1 handful

2. Kale. This food is not only super-trendy, it is filled with nutrients. One cup of kale is an excellent source of vitamin A, vitamin C, and vitamin K, magnesium, and a good source of fiber. Suggested serving: 1-2 cups of raw kale for salads and juicing

3. Oysters. "Oysters are incredibly low in calories and decrease inflammation," says New York nutritionist Bonnie Taub-Dix, R.D. and author of *Read It before You Eat It*. Oysters are heart-healthy and contribute to that great feeling after eating, because they improve overall circulation. Oysters are also very high in essential nutrients like omega-3 fatty acids. And, of course, they have long been considered an aphrodisiac. They are a great source of zinc, vitamin B12, and regulates mood and memory. Suggested serving: 6-12 oysters

4. Coffee. Coffee is practically a magic bean, when it comes to mood lifting. The caffeine in coffee can boost mental focus and alertness. It is said to help athletic performance, protect against Type 2 diabetes, and decrease the risk of depression. Suggested serving: Coffee has about 150 mg of caffeine per cup (consume it once a day, at the time you want to be most alert)

5. Dark Chocolate. Dark chocolate not only provides immediate eating pleasure, but it has a high percentage of cacao or cocoa, which has more antioxidant power than many other foods. Suggested serving: 2-4 small squares a day

Remember that a healthy life style includes a positive mental attitude. We just looked at several important factors in gaining and maintaining a positive mental attitude – your "why" statement, positive thinking, mediation, aromatherapy, yoga, sleep, and happy foods. In our next chapter, we will discuss healthy eating.

# Healthy Eating

*So whether you eat or drink or whatever you do, do it all for the glory of God.*

*I Corinthians 10:31 (NIV)*

Having discussed the importance of a positive mental attitude, we turn our focus to healthy eating. In this chapter, we will discuss the following topics:

- Macronutrients and micronutrients
- Clean eating
- Hanger
- Mindful eating

Why is what you eat so important? As a wellness coach, I have learned that there are five characteristics of healthy eating – adequacy, balance, calorie control, moderation, and variety. Adequacy means that you get enough food to provide essential nutrients and calories. Balance is avoiding overemphasis of any food type or nutrient. Calorie control is having enough calories to supply you with the proper amount of energy, but not too much. Avoid excessive amounts of salt, fat, or sugar. Variety is all about consuming different foods.

# Macronutrients and Micronutrients

Macronutrients are carbohydrates, proteins, and unsaturated fats. Vitamins and minerals are micro-nutrients. All nutrients play different but vital roles in our health and wellbeing. Relying on clean eating, (i.e., we will discuss this in the next section), is the best way to get a good combination of macronutrients and micronutrients.

**Carbohydrates.** Carbohydrates are one of the three macronutrients in food, and you need them for energy and fuel. When you eat carbohydrates, they get broken down into sugars (i.e., glucose, fructose, and galactose) and are either quickly used for energy or are stored as glycogen, in your liver and muscles for use later.

According to Shape.com, "How fast they get broken down depends on the type of carb you eat. Simple carbohydrates quickly get broken down into your bloodstream and give you a supercharge of energy, but leave you at a low later on. Classic examples are fruit juice, white bread, white rice, cereals with little fiber, bagels, and candy. Complex carbohydrates contain less sugar and also have fiber, so they are broken down at a slower rate. These carbohydrates include fruits, vegetables, and whole grains. These are the ones that also help keep your cholesterol levels and weight under control."

According to Shape.com, a person should have about 50 to 60 percent of their calories from carbohydrates. For example, if you consume 1,500 calories a day, 50% would be 750 calories from carbohydrates. Since one gram of carbohydrate equals 4 calories, you can have 187 grams of carbohydrates a day. Low carb diets, consuming 100-150 grams of carbohydrates a day work for some people.

*Fruits and Vegetables.* Eating a variety of fruits and vegetables (i.e., 2 cups of fruit and 2 ½ cups of vegetables) gives your body vitamins, minerals, and phytochemicals (i.e., pigment found in plant based foods that is believe to slow the aging process, boost the immune function, decrease blood pressure and cholesterol, prevent cataracts, have positive effects on cancer, and make the heart and circulatory system stronger). Aim to have at least three different colors of fruits and vegetables daily.

Keep a variety of fresh, frozen, and canned fruit and vegetables in that order to choose from. Fresh is the best, but when not available choose frozen, because the freezing process normally happens immediately after harvest. If you must use can fruit and vegetables, rinse the water off the vegetables to remove the salt. Also choose fruit with natural juice or light syrup.

**Protein.** Protein contains building blocks (i.e., amino acids) used in making enzymes, hormones, antibodies, and neurotransmitters. These building blocks are used to aid growth and body maintenance. It is useful for muscle, hair, skin, organ, tissue repair, and strengthening your immune system. Protein is not just about steak or cheese. Vegetarian sources include beans, tofu, other soy products, quinoa, lentils, and eggs. If you eat meat, have it no more than three times a week. Try to incorporate fish at least twice a week. Dairy products such as milk, cheese, and yogurt are another great source of protein. You should be careful if you are lactose intolerance.

How much protein should you have? The amount of protein a person should consume rages from .5 grams per pound of their body weight to 1.5 grams per pound. The .5 grams is for the average healthy sedentary adult who does not work out and has no fitness goals. The 1.5 grams range is for the average healthy adult who is exercising and has some fitness goals like losing weight and/or muscle toning.[14]

To be clear, if you weigh 150 lbs. then you can consume 75 grams of protein a day to satisfy the .5 grams per pound criteria. You can consume 225 grams to satisfy the 1.5 grams per pound criteria.

**Fats.** Fat is an important macronutrient. It is needed for organ cushioning, vitamin absorption, and growth. According to heart.org, there are four major dietary fats in the foods we eat. The first two types of fats are saturated and trans fats. Saturated fats are typically solid at room temperature. It is possible that eating foods that contain saturated fats will raise cholesterol in your blood. You can find this fat mainly from animal sources, including meat and dairy products. The following are examples:

- fatty beef
- lamb
- pork
- poultry with skin

- lard and cream
- butter
- cheese and
- other dairy products made from whole or reduced-fat (2 percent) milk.

There are two types of trans fats - natural and artificial. Natural trans fats are found in the organs of animals. Artificial trans fats are found in processed foods. Food companies began using hydrogenated *oil* to help increase shelf life and save costs. Hydrogenation is a process in which a liquid unsaturated fat is turned into a solid fat by adding hydrogen. During this processing, a type of fat called trans fat is made. Companies put partially hydrogenated oils in foods because they are easy to use, inexpensive to produce and last a long time. Trans fats give foods a desirable taste and texture. Trans fats should be eaten in moderation, because trans fat raises your LDL ("bad") cholesterol and lowers your HDL ("good") cholesterol.

Heart.org goes on to share that there are two types of good fats – monounsaturated and polyunsaturated.[15] Both of these fats/oils are typically liquid at room temperature but start to turn solid when chilled.

Monounsaturated fats can help reduce bad cholesterol levels in your blood which can lower your risk of heart disease and stroke. They also provide nutrients to help develop and maintain your body's cells. Oils rich in monounsaturated fats also contribute an important antioxidant to the diet called vitamin E. The following are examples:

- olive oil
- canola oil
- peanut oil
- safflower oil
- sesame oil
- avocados
- peanut butter
- nuts and seeds

Nutritionist say that polyunsaturated fat decreases your LDL-cholesterol and HDL-cholesterol. When too much polyunsaturated fat is consumed, the HDL-cholesterol or the good cholesterol is negatively affected. The following are examples:

- soybean oil
- corn oil

- sunflower oil
- fatty fish such as salmon, mackerel, herring, and trout
- walnuts
- sunflower seeds
- tofu
- soybeans

The Dietary Guidelines for Americans gives the following recommendations for fats in the diet:

1. Consume less than 10% of calories from saturated fatty acids and less than 300 mg/day of cholesterol, and keep trans fat consumption as low as possible.

2. Keep total fat intake between 20% to 35% of calories, with most fats coming from sources of polyunsaturated and monounsaturated fat, such as fish, nuts, and vegetable oils.

3. When selecting and preparing meat, poultry, dry beans, and milk or milk products, make choices that are lean, low fat, or fat free.

Micronutrients are not the same as macronutrients (protein, carbohydrates and fat). They are comprised of vitamins and minerals which are required in small quantities, but they are not produced by the body. You must eat a variety of food to get the vitamins and minerals needed for normal metabolism, growth and physical well-being. Consult your family doctor to determine if you will benefit from a supplement.

Even though the body only requires tiny amounts of micronutrients, a micronutrient deficiency can cause serious problems. Sharon Kirby says in her article, What Are Health Benefits of Micronutrients?, that vitamin A, folic acid, iodine, iron and zinc deficiencies are prevalent worldwide and can have grave consequences for children, pregnant women and women of childbearing age.[16] The following is more information from the Webmd about these micronutrients and how the deficiency can affect the body:

- Vitamin A. Vitamin A, or retinol, is a fat-soluble vitamin needed for good vision and healthy skin, teeth, bones and soft tissue. Vitamin A is present in red meat, liver, kidney, fish oil, eggs, dairy products and fortified foods. When you eat yellow and orange fruits and vegetables (i.e., green leafy vegetables) the body converts the Beta-carotene into vitamin. Vitamin A deficiency can lead to vision problems and increase the likelihood of infections.

- Folic Acid. Folic acid, also known as folate or vitamin B-9, is a water-soluble vitamin important for DNA, cell growth, the formation of body tissues and the prevention of birth defects. Folic acid is found in green leafy vegetables such as spinach and kale, orange juice and fortified breakfast cereals. Folic acid deficiency can lead to anemia and birth defects.

- Iodine. Iodine is an essential mineral needed to make thyroid hormones, which are needed for healthy growth. Iodine is found in table salt, but it is also found in fish, kelp or seaweed, garlic, sesame seeds, spinach and squash. An iodine deficiency can cause delayed growth and development, fatigue, weight gain, sensitivity to fluctuating temperatures and dry skin.

- Iron. Iron is an essential mineral needed for the formation of hemoglobin, a protein present in red blood cells that transports oxygen around the body. Iron can be found in red meat, liver, poultry, salmon, tuna, egg yolk, dried beans, dried fruits, whole grains, nuts and green leafy vegetables. An iron deficiency can lead to iron deficiency anemia.

- Zinc. Zinc is an essential mineral required for normal growth and development, healthy skin, infection prevention and wound healing. Zinc is found in red meat, poultry, oysters, beans, nuts, whole grains and fortified breakfast cereals. A zinc deficiency might cause delayed growth and development in children and adolescents, hair loss, diarrhea, delayed wound healing, loss of appetite and weight loss.

**Calorie Intake.** It is common knowledge among fitness experts that your calorie intake should be about 10 calories per pound of the weight that you want to be. For example, if you want to weigh 150 pounds, you would consume about 1,500 calories a day. This assumes moderate activity. If you live a very sedentary lifestyle, you may want to consume eight calories per pound. If you are very active, you may be able to get away with 12 calories per pound.

Because 3,500 calories make a pound of body weight, you can lose one pound a week, by consuming 500 calories less a day than you need to consume. If you add extra activity to your lower calorie intake, you can speed the weight lost up.

## Clean Eating

Clean eating is a modern phrase which essentially means eating foods that are as close to their natural state as possible. I really enjoyed the simple way dummies.com described clean eating. They said to eat whole foods (i.e., foods straight from the farm: whole fruits and vegetables, whole grains, grass-fed and free-range meats, low fat dairy products, unsalted nuts, and seeds); avoid processed foods (i.e., any food that has more than one ingredient, and ingredients that you cannot pronounce); eliminate refined sugar (i.e., try other sweeteners); eat five or six small meals a day (i.e., this can help speed up your metabolism and reduce the chances that you will eat foods that are not so good for you); cook your own meals (i.e., clean and whole foods need little preparation); and combine protein with carbohydrates (i.e., this will help you create satisfying and balanced snacks and meals).[17]

**So what might a day's healthy, clean eating look like?** The following is a sample clean eating meal plan:

Breakfast. Two poached eggs on a slice of buttered wholegrain bread and some chopped tomatoes.

Mid-morning snack. Apple or other piece of fruit, served with a small handful of raw unsalted nuts.

Lunch. Tuna salad, made with canned tuna, 2-3 tablespoons of cooked navy beans, salad dressing, salad leaves, chopped cucumber, and plain yogurt with berries.

Dinner. Roasted chicken thighs or legs, a roasted sweet potato, and steamed broccoli.

Evening snack. Melon, slice of whole grain bread with peanut butter, and a cup of skim milk.

**Weight Loss Foods.** The following list of foods have proven to help burn calories and fight the hunger that can lead to eating less healthy and more fattening foods[18]:

- Low-fat milk, yogurt, and cottage cheese. According to experts, people on lower-calorie diets who had three to four servings of dairy foods (especially low fat Greek yogurt – 12 grams of protein) each day lost more weight than those who ate a low-dairy diet with the same number of calories.
- Berries. Fiber is a big part of weight loss, because it helps you feel full sooner and stays in your stomach longer. Berries (i.e., strawberries, blackberries, and blueberries) are full of fiber (as much as 8 grams) and are low in carbs.
- High-fiber cereals. These have fewer calories than eggs, bacon, donuts, and muffins. The fiber helps keep you feeling full all morning, so you are less likely to need a snack before lunch. Also, fiber helps keep insulin,

which our bodies use to control starch and sugar, at the right level. This in turn slows fat storage.

- Oranges, grapefruits, lemons, and limes. According to health experts, Vitamin C helps burn fat faster and makes losing weight easier. One study found that people who ate half a grapefruit with each meal for 12 weeks lost about 3.6 pounds. The study suggests this Vitamin C-packed citrus fruit lowers insulin, or "blood sugar," which in turn helps weight loss. Remember if you are taking medicine, check with your doctor, before eating grapefruit, since some medicines do not combine well with it.

- Green tea. The caffeine in green tea is a natural way to help burn more calories, speed up the heart rate, and free fatty acids stored in the body, so they are more ready for energy use. Also, green tea has something called ECGC, which may help speed the way your body uses food, by speeding up the nervous system.

- Water. Some researchers say hunger pangs are thirst in disguise. The signs of dehydration look like the signs of hunger - weakness, tiredness, crankiness, etc. The old "drink 8 glasses a day" rule still holds true for making sure our systems are running smoothly and getting rid of anything that should not be in our bodies.

- Salmon, tuna, and sardines. These fish are said to have high amounts of Omega-3 fatty acids, which help burn calories. It is said that fish oil can boost peoples' fat-burning levels, by as much as 400 calories a day.
- Lean beef, chicken, and turkey. These foods help speed up calorie use and burn more fat.
- Spicy peppers. Jalapeños, chili peppers, etc. contain a chemical that speeds up the heart rate and helps the body burn more fat.
- Apples and pears. Women who ate three small apples or pears a day lost more weight on a low-calorie diet than women who did not eat these fruits.
- Soup. A Penn State University study shows soup is very good for controlling hunger, because it is made up of a satisfying blend of liquid and solid food.

- Broccoli. This vegetable is high in calcium and in Vitamin C, which helps the body take in more calcium, and it only has 20 calories per cup.

## Hanger

After finishing a 15K run, I heard a young lady say an interesting word, "hangry." She said, "I should have eaten a better breakfast, so that I wouldn't be so 'hangry'." I thought she made the word up, until my insurance (Humana) sent me an email asking do I sometimes get "hangry?" Well, hangry is when your blood sugar drops so low that it makes you unable to do normal functions. You will find yourself both hungry and angry. This is not a great combination.

The Humana.com health article, "How to Beat Hanger," states that the dropping of the sugar level affects your hormones and mood. Deborah Levy, MS, RD, says, "When you eat, the body breaks down the sugars and starches into glucose to fuel the body's cells."[19] A drop in your blood sugar, or glucose level, which is the body's main source of energy, means a drop in your vitality and self-control, fueling not only those moody food-seeking binges but a cranky outlook on a perfectly fine day.

She goes on to say, "Not everyone experiences it; some people are more susceptible than others." Blood sugar can drop because you have not eaten anything in a while or you have not eaten the right things. Levy says "We're not sure why hangar happens to some people, perhaps they have more stressors, their mood is spotty to begin with, or they're just sensitive to it. Then they eat something like a plain bagel with butter for breakfast and their blood sugar, which should be around 75-100mg/dL, rises rapidly and crashes just as quickly dropping very low to something like 55 mg/dL causing hangar."

The more you skip meals and the more you eat simple carbohydrates, the worse you feel hanger, because simple carbohydrates and all that sugar moves through the bloodstream quickly. Deborah Levy says, "Hanger is both physiological and emotional. It's physiological because you're hungry, and it's emotional because now you're angry."

Levy gives the following few tips to keep a person from getting hangry:

1. Proper combination of fruit, vegetables, whole grains, and protein. Levy believes that a person should have a balanced ratio of protein, whole grains, and colorful produce that helps energy and fuel release like a time capsule vitamin. Research shows whole grains give immediate energy, protein provides staying power to feel full longer, and water and fiber in veggies give the needed vitamins and minerals for optimal physical and mental functioning.

2. Eat on a schedule with four to five hours between meals. Other fitness experts recommend eating three to four hours between meals. She goes on to say, snacking between meals is allowed. Make sure you are combining your food properly.

3. Remember to eat slow carbs. Levy gives a great example of the difference. Fast or simple carbs like donuts and candy bars are like the biggest rollercoaster you have ever ridden. You go all the way to the top and then fall all the way down at breakneck speed. Slow or complex carbs like whole grains, fruit, vegetables, and proteins are like a baby roller coaster. You go up slowly

for a while, linger at the top, and then slide down more gingerly.

**Hanger Meal Plan.** The following is a meal plan to help you beat hanger (taken from Humana.com):

Breakfast: oatmeal with blueberries and chia or flax seeds; or breakfast bar and a banana; or bran cereal and melon

Lunch: turkey sandwich on whole grain bread with carrot sticks; or chicken whole grain wrap with broccoli and red peppers; or vegetable salad with tuna and whole grain roll

Snacks: hardboiled egg with whole wheat crackers and an apple; or cheese stick, handful of grapes, and a couple of whole grain crackers

Dinner: brown rice, chicken breast, and asparagus spears; or quinoa, lean beef tips, and green beans.

## Mindful Eating

Mindful eating is being more aware of your eating habits, the sensations you experience when you eat, and the thoughts and emotions that you have about food. It is more about how you eat than what you eat.

Caloriecount.com says, we must eat with intention and attention. What is eating with intention? It simply means be purposeful. Ask yourself am I hungry, what does my body need to be healthy, and do you feel better after eating?

Eating with attention means devoting your full interest to what you are eating. This can be done by eliminating distractions (e.g., T.V., newspapers, electronic devices, etc.), using your five senses as you eat, and listening to your body to see if you are truly hungry.

## Shopping tips

The following are some tips for shopping:

1. Try writing out your list the day before and plan all of your meals. Write out your requirements, and make sure you give yourself a reward, if you stick to it (i.e., a nice warm bath perhaps).

2. Do not do your shopping, while you are hungry. Think about all those delicious

smells. Eat a meal or at least a snack before you go.

3. Give yourself a limited time. Force yourself to be in and out in half an hour. That means you will need to stick to that list, and rushing from aisle to aisle helps you fit in a bit of exercise.

4. Shop later in the day. If you shop later on in the evening, supermarkets often mark down fresh produce such as fish, meat, fruits, and vegetables. By freezing what you do not cook, you can save a few dollars.

5. Try grocery shopping online, if possible. It stops you from falling for offers, and it is more likely to make you stick to a list (this obviously is not possible in all areas).

**Eating to Improve Exercising.** Per my study of an article, "Eat Like an Olympian,"[20] I would recommend that you eat a snack 1-2 hours before exercising. Fruits and vegetables, whole grains, and lean protein should be your focus. I also recommend that thirty to 60 minutes after finishing your workout, eat carbohydrate-rich foods with some protein. Think about a peanut butter sandwich (half or whole), carton of chocolate milk, or a bowl of cereal with milk or yogurt.

In this chapter, we have discussed macro and micronutrients, clean eating, hanger, and mindful eating. You may not change everything today. But you owe it to yourself to make a least one or two improvements today related to your eating. In the next chapter, we will talk about physical activity.

# Physical Activity

"So I run straight to the goal with purpose in every step. I fight to win. I'm not just shadow-boxing or playing around. Like an athlete I punish my body, treating it roughly, training it to do what it should, not what it wants to. Otherwise I fear that after enlisting others for the race, I myself might be declared unfit and ordered to stand aside." 1 Corinthians 9:26-27 (TLB)

"Exercise is to your body what fine-tuning is to the engine of your car."
Cornell Chin, *Celebrity Body for Cheap*

"Don't make exercise a half-hearted endeavor! Set goals, create a plan, and then execute it. Don't be afraid to pay for help. Beliefnet.com[21]

Having looked at healthy eating, we now focus on physical activity. In this chapter, we will discuss the following:

- Benefits of exercising
- Types of exercises
- Amount of exercise
- Warning signs
- Gym membership
- Home exercise routines

# Benefits of Exercising

The following are some benefits of exercising:

- It helps to strengthen the body (e.g., heart, lungs, and muscles).
- It helps to control and reduce weight, by burning calories and reducing fat.
- It helps to reduce the risk of several diseases like type 2 diabetes, heart disease, high blood pressure, and stroke.
- It helps you look great and improve your quality of life.
- It helps you with your mood. Exercising produces endorphins – chemicals that are naturally released during and after exercise that helps relieve pain, lift mood, and control stress.

## Types of Exercises

According to the fitness community, there are four components of exercising.

1. Cardio-Respiratory Endurance. This is the ability to deliver oxygen and nutrients to tissues and to remove wastes, over sustained periods of time.

Long runs and swims are among the methods used in measuring this component.

2. Muscular Strength. This is the ability of your muscles to exert force for a brief period of time. Upper body strength, for example, can be measured by various weightlifting exercises.

3. Muscular Endurance. This is the ability of your muscle, or a group of muscles, to sustain repeated contractions or to continue applying force against a fixed object. Push-ups are often used to test endurance of chest, arm, and shoulder muscles.

4. Flexibility. This is the ability to move your joints and use muscles through their full range of motion. The sit and reach test is a good measure of flexibility of the lower back and the backs of the upper legs.[22]

## Amount of Exercise

To develop or maintain a healthy life style, it is important to do aerobic activity to get your heart beating faster. The following is a partial list of aerobic activities:

- Dancing
- Biking
- Sports (e.g., basketball, football, soccer)
- Walking fast
- Water aerobics
- Jogging
- Swimming
- Chair exercising
- Zumba
- Tennis
- Gardening
- Jump rope
- Boxing

For most healthy adult, the U.S. Government guidelines advise that a person striving to maintain their weight should aim for at least 30 minutes on most days of the week. If a person is interested in losing weight or keeping weight loss off, they should aim for at least 60 to 90 minutes on most days. It is important to note that you can do 10 minutes at a time, instead of all 30-90 minutes of exercise at one time.

**Intensity.** After determining how much exercise you need, understanding intensity is important. The book Practical Aerobic Conditioning says intensity is "the amount or degree of effort involved in an exercise or movement." The simplified method to determine your training heart rate range is determined as follows:

1. Determine your maximum heart range (MHR). This is done by taking the maximum number of times the heart can beat in a minute (220) and subtract your age. For example, a healthy 50 year old female would use this formula, 220-50= 170 MHR.

2. Decide what training heart rate zone (i.e., the range you need to be in for cardiorespiratory training to take place). The healthy 50 year old female may want to use the recommended range of 55% to 90% of her MHR. This is determined by multiplying the MHR by .55 or by .90. Let's assume this person has been exercising for a while. She may periodically hit the 90% higher limit of her MHR while exercising. This will make her heart rate reading 153. After cooling down (i.e., 3-5 minutes) the heart rate reading should be less than 55% of the MHR or less than 93.5.

3. Another way to measure intensity is by using the "Rate of Perceived Exertion."

"Perceived exertion is how hard you feel like your body is working. It is based on the physical sensations a person experiences during physical activity, including increased heart rate, increased respiration or breathing rate, increased sweating, and muscle fatigue. Although this is a subjective measure, a person's exertion rating may provide a fairly good estimate of the actual heart rate during physical activity."[23] Dr. Gunnar Borg, a Swedish professor emeritus of Perception and Psychophysics at Stockholm University teaches that you should self-monitoring how hard your body is working so you adjust the intensity of the activity by speeding up or slowing down. The Borg Rating of Perceived Exertion (RPE) scale ranges from 6 to 20, where 6 means "no exertion at all" and 20 means "maximal exertion." To calculate your heart rate using this method, add a zero to what your RPE. For example, if during your workout you perceive you are working at a 15 your heart rate is 150 beats per minute. Be mindful these numbers are what you perceive.

4. An easy way to determine your intensity level is to buy a good sports watch that monitors your heart rate.

We now move from how much activity you need to warning signs.

## Warning Signs

I wrote in my article, "Physical Exercise: Three Warnings,"[24] that physical exercise is good for you but can lead to injuries. Below are three warnings to be familiar with regarding exercising too much.

1. Unrealistic goals. You should exercise to lose weight. However, some people over exercise to speed up weight loss. Television, magazines, internet, billboards, radio, and the like and then our family, friends, and familiar have lead many into having unrealistic goals. Some think they can lose a clothing size in one week, if they start exercising two or three times a day every day. It is recommended by About.com that a healthy adult should engage in moderate exercise at least thirty minutes five times a week.[25]

Remember, if it took you months to put on that extra 20 pounds, it will take time to lose it. Be realistic in your expectations, and it will take away some of your stress.

2. Your body needs rest. The body needs to do some form of exercise, but it also needs rest. Over exercising can lead to injuries like fractures and muscle strains.

3. Fads do not work. There are many fairy tale workouts and diets that just do not work. Some people think that just lifting weights will produce a healthy body. Others think cardio alone will produce a healthy body. Others think dieting will produce the healthy body they are looking for. It takes diet and exercise to produce a healthy body.

If you look in some people's basement, it will look like a sports store. They go from one fad to another. They spend so much time and money on products that do not produce speedy results. Once again, it takes time and work to stay healthy. It is important to do a little at a time and then add on as you feel comfortable. Dr. Baines shares some great insight on exercising on his website, GettingInShapeAfter40.com.[26]

Understanding warning signs will help you as you look into "do you need a gym membership"?

## Do You Need a Gym Membership?

Having a gym membership is helpful to some and wasteful to others. It is helpful if a person goes and use the equipment (e.g., treadmills, bikes, weights, etc.), take classes (e.g., group classes, swim, etc.), or engage with others in the gym. To this person, going to the gym may be part of their weekly routine, and it is enjoyable to them.

Others may see the gym as boring, time consuming, and a waste of money. Some enjoy being outside or exercising in their homes. A person can enjoy a healthy lifestyle without a gym.

Just remember to be active. Sitting for long periods of time can lead to obesity, weakness of the buttock muscles, lower back problems, tightness of the hamstring, and other health related issues.

Note the following ways of being active without the gym, per the American Heart Association:

- Stand as much as you can.
- Walk to tell co-workers messages.
- Be an **in**efficient house keeper. Instead of piling your belongings into one batch to take upstairs or into another room, take things in small amounts, so there are more trips and activity.
- Walk where you can.
- Dance to music on the radio.
- Gardening.
- Take a brisk walk (or run) for 20-30 minutes four or five times a week.
- Exercise to a DVD.
- High Intensity Interval Training (or HIIT for short). This is when you exercise very intensively for a short period, say 45 seconds to a minute, then walk or rest for a period (again, say 45 seconds to a minute) and repeat several times.

Determining whether you need a gym membership is important. In the next section you will be given some exercises to do at home.

## Home Exercise Routines

When working out at home, be conscious of injury prevention. Listen to your body. If it hurts, stop doing that. If it is too difficult, make it easier. Another great way to prevent injuries is to rest the body, when needed.

Cardio workouts can be done consistently for five to six days. However, it is recommended that you rest a day in between your weight routines.

Here is a suggested way to get your exercising in and rest your body. Monday through Friday do at least thirty minutes of a moderate to intense cardio routine. A moderate routine may be walking in place, kicking, dancing, or other activities that warm your body. An intense cardio routine can be something like doing jumping jacks, jogging in place, or any other activity that can make you feel hot. Do your weights at least two days on opposite days. Tuesdays and Thursdays can be used as weight days and Saturdays can be a day for extras (cardio and/or weights).

I recommend you start out with something as simple as marching in place for 10 minute bouts. Working continuously for 10 minutes and doing it a couple more times throughout the day is about as effective as doing one 30 minute session. Below I share a routine that I found to be effective with my clients.

This exercise routine can be done at home or at the gym, alone or with a buddy, fast or slow. The routine is design to be basic, so that you can add your personal touch to it. Try to do the routine for at least 20 minutes and at least three to four times a week.

## Basic Exercise Routine

The basic exercise routine below is from my article, An Easy Exercise Routine for You. See the article for details on how to perform the exercises.[27]

- *March in place for two minutes*. Start by standing upright with arms at your side, alternate picking up knees and swinging opposite arms. Make sure your abs are tight (i.e., your stomach is sucked in). Relax your shoulders, push out your chest, pick your chin up, and look ahead. Imagine you are a soldier in a parade of honor guards (smile). This exercise warms up the body and elevates your heart rate.

The following exercises can be done for a count of 32 then for a count of 16 and then for a count of 8. If you need less time doing the exercises, cut the count down in half (i.e., a count of 16, then a count of 8, followed by a count of 4).

- **Arm Rotations.** Start by standing upright with your legs shoulder width apart. Extend both arms to the side, and twirl slowly. Make sure your abs are tight, your shoulders are relaxed, push out your chest, pick your chin up, and look ahead. Control your rotations and focus on muscles that you are working. This exercise works especially your shoulders, triceps, and biceps. The smaller the move the more difficult the exercise becomes.
- **Jumping Jacks.** Standing upright with arms to your side, begin with a jump with legs shoulder with apart and both arms going over your head. Jump again, and bring in both legs and arms back down to your sides. Make sure your abs are tight, your shoulders are relaxed, push out your chest, pick your chin up, and look ahead. Control your arm raises, because you can possible damage your rotor cuff, if you swing your arms uncontrolled over your head. When

you jump, try to land on the balls of your feet. If you have pain in the front of your legs, it is suggested that you land with your knees slightly bent and land with your feet softly on the floor.

- **Twist.** This exercise is a great exercise for the abs and back (i.e., your core). Start off by standing upright with a towel in your hands, with elbows slightly bent or elbows bent without a towel, and fist to the front and chest high. Stand with legs shoulder width apart, with your back straight, your abs tight, your shoulders relaxed, looking ahead with your chest and chin up, begin twisting left to right. It is important to keep your hips and head stationary and work your midsection or core.

- **Crunches.** If you want to work your stomach or abs, lay on your back, on the floor. Bend your knees and place your hands behind your head or on your chest, whichever is most comfortable for you. The simplest way to do this exercise is simply suck your stomach in and roll forward. Be careful not to pull the neck, let the abs do the work, even if the movement is small. Try to push up towards the ceiling, and hold for a second at the top. Make sure you breathe out, when you crunch up, and breathe in, when you go down.

- **Plank.** Another name for this exercise is the bridge. Lay flat on your stomach, on the floor, with your elbows bent close to your chest and your toes on the floor. Push up with your elbows and toes, and make sure your back is straight, by sucking in your abs. Align your body in a neutral position, by looking down at the floor. This exercise works the arms, chest, back, abs, glut (i.e., buttock), and legs.

- **Bird Dog.** Start this exercise by getting on all four limbs, on the floor. Extend your right arm and left leg, and hold for 32 counts. Switch sides and extend the left arm and right leg. Hold for 32 counts. This exercise is great for the arms, glut, legs, back, and abs. Make sure your body is neutrally aligned, by looking towards the floor to alleviate neck pain.

- Repeat the routine as time allows.

Aim to do what you can, and push yourself a little more each time, by adding more energy and time to your exercise routine.

## Simple Exercise Routine

As you get stronger and have more endurance, try this other exercise routine that I recommend to my clients.

- Warm-up and stretch for five minutes. Keep your knees slightly bent, stomach tight, and back straight the entire routine. Remember to breathe in your nose and out your mouth.

- March in place for 16 counts (knees high, swing arms forward and back).

- 16 Heel digs (leg goes forward, heel touches the floor, toes are up, make a muscle with your opposite arm, and switch leg and arms)

- 16 Kick and punch (kick leg out, punch out with the opposite arm, and switch leg and arms)

- 16 Hamstring curls (curl your leg as though you are trying to touch your "bottom," pull your arms back and switch legs)

- Step to right and then to the left for 32 counts.

- Lunge your right leg to the front with arms up, breathe in and blow it out as you reach towards your toes, and switch. Do on both sides twice.

- Stretch up to the right (legs are shoulder width apart) and then to the left. Do on both sides twice.

- Arms over your head. Breathe in and reach for the floor as you breathe out. Do twice.

**Let's move (5 minutes)**

- March in place for 16 counts (knees high, swing arms forward and back).

- 16 Heel digs (leg goes forward, heel touches the floor, toes are up, make a muscle with your opposite arm, and switch leg and arms)

- 16 Kick and punch (kick right leg out, punch out with the left arm, and switch leg and arms)

- 16 Hamstring curls (curl your leg as though you are trying to touch your "bottom," pull your arms back and switch legs)

- Step side to side and hold arms out to the side like you are flying - 16 count.

- 16 Jacks (leg to the side with heel on the floor, arms go over head, switch legs)

If time allows, repeat this entire "let's move" twice - smile.

**Cool down and Stretch (5 minutes)**
- March in place for 16 counts (knees high, swing arms forward and back)
- 16 Heel digs (leg goes forward, heel touches the floor, toes are up, make a muscle with your opposite arm, and switch leg and arms)
- 16 Hamstring curls (curl your leg as though you are trying to touch your "bottom," pull your arms back and switch legs)
- Step side to side for 16
- Right leg lunge to the front with arms up, breathe in and blow it out as you reach towards your toes, and switch. Do on both sides twice.
- Stretch up to the right (legs are shoulder width apart) and then to the left. Do on both sides twice.
- Arms over your head. Breathe in and reach for the floor as you breathe out. Do this twice.

In this chapter, we have discussed the types of exercises, benefits of exercising, amount of exercise, warning signs, do you need a gym membership, and home exercise routines. I would urge you to listen to your body and doctor. As you get started with wherever you are, add on to your routine as you are able. Reading this book is a great start, but you have to move your body. In our next chapter, we will look at "changes in hormones and sickness."

# Changes in Hormones and Sickness

*"For I the LORD do not change; therefore you, O children of Jacob, are not consumed."*
Malachi 3:6 (RSV)

Having looked at physical activity, we now focus on changes in hormones and sickness. In this chapter, we will discuss the following:

- Hormones
- Endorphins
- Hypertension
- Diabetes

## Hormones

**Female Menopause.** I believe most of us have heard about women experiencing menopause. According to the Mayo Clinic, menopause is defined as happening 12 months after a woman experiences their last menstrual period. It can happen in their 40s or 50s, but in the United States the average age is 51.[28]

Some reasons women experience menopause are aging (i.e., ovaries start making less hormones - estrogen and progesterone); total hysterectomy (i.e., removal of both the uterus and ovaries); chemotherapy and radiation; and genetics (i.e., your family may have a history of early onset of menopause or what some call premature menopause).

Estrogen and progesterone are important in women health. These hormones are useful with ovulation, menstruation, skin, bone, breast tissue, the uterine lining, blood vessels, and tissues of the breast, vagina, uterus, and other organs.

The following are signs and symptoms that a woman may be going through menopause:

- Irregular periods
- Vaginal dryness
- Hot flashes
- Night sweats
- Sleep problems
- Mood changes
- Weight gain and slowed metabolism
- Thinning hair and dry skin
- Loss of breast fullness

## Male Menopause

According to the medical community, men also experience changes with their hormones. WebMD says there is debate in the medical community whether men actually experience male menopause. It does say some doctors refer to this problem as androgen - decline in the aging male or what some people call low testosterone. [29] [30]

Livestrong.com says testosterone is necessary for muscle and bone strength, sperm production, and sex drive. It also helps regulate fat distribution and the production of red blood cells. Testosterone may even improve mood, memory, and energy levels.

It is very important for a man to have his annual exam and learn his numbers. The bottom of a man's normal total testosterone range is about 300 nanograms per deciliter (ng/dL). The upper limit is about 800ng/dL depending on the lab.

Below is a list that WedMd.com provided as signs and symptoms that a man may be going through male menopause or experiencing low testosterone:

- Low sex drive
- Difficulty in having an erection
- Low semen volume
- Hair loss
- Fatigue and lack of energy
- Muscle loss
- Increase in body fat
- Mood change

When checking the levels of testosterones, a lower than normal score on a blood test can be caused by a number of conditions, including the following:

- Injury to the testicles
- Testicular cancer or treatment for testicular cancer
- Hormonal disorders
- Infection
- HIV/AIDS
- Chronic liver or kidney disease
- Type 2 diabetes
- Obesity
- Medicines
- Genetics

The following are some ways to naturally boost low testosterone:

- Get more sleep
- Lose excess weight

- Eat more zinc – red meat, poultry, nuts, beans, oysters, crabs, lobster, and whole grain
- Ease off the sugar
- Exercise

**Endorphins.** Endorphins are natural chemicals made by your body. When they are released, they have a powerful, positive effect on your emotional well-being. "Endorphins are a group of peptide hormones that occur naturally in the brain that, when released, increase your body's threshold for pain and affect the way you feel emotionally. Endorphins are chemically very much like morphine. There are a few things you can do to possibly release endorphins and increase your mood." Ehow.com says to, "Exercise hard. Most athletes will tell you of a 'runner's high' that they sometimes feel when they push their bodies to the limit. Endorphins are released when you are involved in strenuous exercise that allows your body to go beyond physical pain and its limitations and it may leave you with a euphoric high." [31]

But exercise is not the only way to release the benefits of endorphins. Here are a few endorphin-releasing activities that do not involve exercise.

- Make things better for someone else. Helping others and being thanked for what you do can help build self-esteem.
- Practice self-discipline. Self-control naturally makes you feel more in control. This is very useful when something in your life is out of your control. Managing what you can about your life, even if it's simply what time you go to bed at night, can help you keep some balance. It can also help you fight off despair, helplessness, and other negative thoughts.
- Learn or discover new things. Take an adult education class, join a book club, or just travel somewhere new. Change really can do you good!
- Enjoy the beauty of nature or art. Studies show that simply walking through a garden can lower blood pressure and stress. Walking through a park or an art gallery works, too. You can also hike or just sit on a beach to lower your blood pressure.

Below is a list of Ehow.com non-exercising endorphin releasing activities:

- Listen to soothing music. It has been found that thirty minutes of listening to classical and instrumental music has released endorphins that have an effect equal to that of the muscle relaxer pill known as Valium.
- Eat some spicy food. Spicy food can cause the brain to release more endorphins.
- Spend some time in the sun. Exposure to light can also cause a release of endorphins.
- Have a healthy sex life. Intense pleasure causes the same effect as intense pain when it comes to endorphins.
- Laugh and cry. Some people claim that laughing hard for ten minutes can give at least two hours of pain-free sleep to those affected by painful illnesses. Some researchers claim that the body releases endorphins to relieve pain, while experiencing the emotion that causes tears.
- Eat something sweet or have something chocolate. These items stimulate your brain's pleasure pathways and causes the release of endorphins. Unfortunately when the short-lived sugar rush is over, so is

the effect of endorphins, and you will be left feeling tired and worn out.

As you go through your season of change, make sure you work on feeling good and taking care of yourself.

## Hypertension

Healthy living is all about making choices that will affect your body in a positive way. But sometimes you do everything right and illness just pops up in your life. In 1989, I was diagnose with hypertension, and in 2004, I was told I had diabetes. Thank God, today both of these illnesses are controlled mainly by diet and exercise.

According to the Centers for Disease Control and Prevention (CDC), high blood pressure (hypertension) is a serious condition that affects one in three adults in the United States. It is called the "silent killer," because people often have no symptoms, yet it can lead to some serious and sometimes even fatal conditions.[32] According to the American Heart Association, a blood pressure reading of less than 120/80 mmHg (millimeters of mercury) is considered normal. When you have high blood pressure, your blood moves through your arteries at a higher pressure, putting more pressure on the delicate tissues and damaging your blood vessels. You are diagnosed with high blood pressure (hypertension), if your blood pressure readings are consistently above 140/90 mmHg.

**What are causes of hypertension?** In most cases of high blood pressure, there is no known cause, according to Healthline.com. This is called primary hypertension. When medical conditions like kidney or heart conditions cause high blood pressure, this is called secondary hypertension. Some medications like birth control pills or over-the-counter cold medicines can cause high blood pressure as well. Blood pressure may or may not return to normal upon discontinuation of the medication.

**High Blood Pressure Risk Factors.** There are many risk factors for high blood pressure. Some factors you cannot change. Like the following:

- Age: Older adults are at greater risk for high blood pressure.

- Gender: Women over 65 are more likely to have higher blood pressure, and men under age 45 are more likely to have high blood pressure than women.
- Race: African-Americans are more likely to have high blood pressure.
- Family history: If your direct family members (i.e., parent or sibling) have high blood pressure, you are more at risk.

Others factors are modifiable based on your lifestyle. Like the following:

- Being overweight
- Not exercising enough
- Eating an unhealthy diet
- Consuming excess salt
- Drinking alcohol
- Smoking
- Sleep apnea
- Stress

If you are able to make a change in your lifestyle that will affect your high blood pressure in a positive way, today is the day to do it.

# Diabetes

Research have shown that diabetes is a disease that causes high blood sugar (glucose) levels in the body, due to defects in insulin production and/or function. Insulin is a hormone released by the pancreas, when we eat food. Insulin allows sugar to go from the blood into the cells. If the cells of the body are not using insulin well, or if the body is unable to make any or enough insulin, sugar builds up in the blood. There are four known types – type 1, type 2, gestational, and prediabetes.

**Type 1 Diabetes.** This is an autoimmune disease and occurs when the body's misdirected immune system attacks and destroys insulin-producing beta cells in the pancreas. The exact cause of type 1 diabetes is not completely understood. Most patients are diagnosed as children or young adults. People with type 1 diabetes must take insulin daily to manage their condition.

**Type 2 Diabetes**. This normally develops gradually with age and is characterized by insulin resistance in the body. For reasons not yet totally understood, the cells of the body stop being able to use insulin effectively. Because of this resistance, the body's fat, liver, and muscle cells are unable to take in and store glucose, which is used for energy. Family history and genetics play a major role in type 2 diabetes. Type 2 diabetes occurs most often in people who are overweight and sedentary.

**Gestational Diabetes.** This is defined as blood-sugar elevation during pregnancy. It is known to affect about three to eight percent of women. Left undiagnosed or untreated, it can lead to problems such as high birth weight and breathing problems for the baby. Gestational diabetes usually resolves in the mother, after the baby is born. But statistics show that women who have gestational diabetes have a much greater chance of developing type 2 diabetes within five to 10 years.

**Prediabetes.** This is thought by some experts to be the first step to type 2 diabetes. This condition is marked by blood sugar levels that are too high to be considered normal but are not yet high enough to be in the range of a typical diabetes diagnosis. Prediabetes increases not only your risk of developing diabetes but also your risk of heart disease and stroke.

According to the American Diabetes Association, the following symptoms of diabetes are typical. However, some people with type 2 diabetes have symptoms so mild that they go unnoticed.

- Urinating often
- Feeling very thirsty
- Feeling very hungry - even though you are eating
- Extreme fatigue
- Blurry vision
- Cuts/bruises that are slow to heal
- Weight loss - even though you are eating more (type 1)
- Tingling, pain, or numbness in the hands/feet (type 2).[33]

In this chapter, we have discussed the following: hormones, female menopause, male menopause, endorphins, hypertension, and diabetes

Changes in hormones, hypertension, and diabetes are some things we may face. Do your best and trust God with the rest.

Before we go to our conclusion, let me challenge you to take the next 30 days and spend 10 minutes a day for at least three days a week to reflect on your health. Prayerfully ask yourself the following five questions and write down your answers:

1. Why does God want me to be healthy?

2. What are some things I am doing well or I am thankful for as it relates to my health?

3. What are some challenges I may be having as it relates to my health?

4. What are some small steps I can make today towards improving my health?

Your answer to question 1 can help you develop your "why" statement. Your answer to question 2 can help you see that you are doing something well and have some things to be thankful for. Your answers to question 3 and 4 can help you get focused on taking small steps towards addressing a challenge or two.

# Conclusion

Healthy living is all about having a positive mindset, engaging in clean eating, being physically active, and managing changes and illnesses, as they happen. We must remember that God is the One who gives us the ability to engage in healthy living. I pray the information that was share will help you become a better you. God desires for us to take care of our bodies which belongs to Him.

I Corinthians 6:19-20 says, [19] Do you not know that your bodies are temples of the Holy Spirit, who is in you, whom you have received from God? You are not your own; [20] you were bought at a price. Therefore honor God with your bodies.

# Book Excerpt: Daniel Fast Diet

**The following is an excerpt from my book, THE DANIEL FAST DIET: A Guide on How Christians can Lose Weight and Gain Spiritual Strength With the Daniel Fast.** [34]

Thank you for taking time out of your busy schedule to read my book, "*Daniel Fast Diet.*" If you are like me, you want to lose weight, but you want it to be easy and fast. Many people do drastic measures and are not successful. They try diets after diets and get more frustrated after each attempt. **This book will show you a way to both lose weight and keep it off.**

This book is written in a way that will give you the bottom line of how to do the Daniel's Fast Diet and then come back to give more details. In Chapter One, we will look at "What is the Daniel's Fast?" Chapter Two is about "How to Do the Daniel's Fast." In Chapter Three, we discuss "Why You Should Do the Daniel's Fast." Chapter Four is all about "Ways to Keep the Weight Off." Chapter Five is about "How Spiritual Strength is Gained

Through the Daniel's Fast." Then there is a bonus chapter on "Recipes for the Daniel's Fast."

Let me encourage you to pray and then read the scriptures. Let God minister to you, as you learn how to lose weight and gain spiritual strength through the Daniel's Fast. I pray God's continual blessings on you, as you begin or continue your journey.

## CHAPTER ONE – WHAT IS THE DANIEL'S FAST DIET?

The Daniel's Fast Diet is simply a way to safely and easily lose weight, by choosing to modify your eating for 21 days. The fast simply involves doing the following things:

1. Eat fruit, vegetables, and lots of legumes (beans and seeds);

2. Drink water for a beverage;

3. Do it for 21 days;

4. Avoid eating meat;

5. Avoid all bread;

6. Avoid sweets; and

7. Avoid artificial, processed, or chemically altered foods.

Many Christians choose to do this fast as a way to get closer to God. I also found this to be a great way to lose some unwanted pounds. It is important to remember that there are different ways to fast. According to WebMd.com, "fasting diets aren't all the same. Some allow only liquids like water, juice, or tea. Others cut calories drastically, but don't completely ban food. And on some plans, you fast every other day."

# About the Author

**Daphene Baines** earned her Master's Degree with an emphasis on family studies from Wright State University (i.e., Fairborn, OH.), in 2004. Since 1990, she has served on various church staffs. She currently serves as a Ministry Assistant at the Southern Baptist Church (i.e., Cincinnati, OH.).

She is certified as a Personal Trainer, Nutrition Consultant, Group Exercise Instructor, and a Life Coach. She uses her training as a Silver Sneakers' Instructor, Diabetes Prevention Specialist, and a Wellness Consultant. She loves to teach health related courses and help individual coaching clients. She loves working with single parent females and the mature adult population.

She loves the Lord and loves to minister to people. She is the lovely wife of Dr. Robert E. Baines, Jr. (see www.Robert-Baines.com). They have two adult daughters (i.e., both in the ministry) and two wonderful grandchildren.

She assists with the managing of the websites at

www.Christian-Living-Site.com

and

www.GettingInShapeAfter40.com

# Helpful Resources and Endnotes

## Resources

- **Your Free Gift -** Dieting Tips: 101 Easy to Follow and Proven Diet Tips That Will Help You Lose Weight in 7 Days (and Thereafter), Without Starving Yourself. *All you have to do is go to the link below and then supply your name and email, in exchange for the booklet, which will be emailed to you in pdf format.*

- American Diabetes Association. http://www.diabetes.org/diabetes-basics/symptoms/?loc=db-slabnav#sthash.8rwPcfS1.dpuf

- http://gettinginshapeafter40.com/go/dieting-tips/

- www.Caloriecounter.com

- www.Christian-Living-Site.com

- http://gettinginshapeafter40.com

- Meditation Techniques: A Step-By-Step Guide on Using Meditation for Anxiety Relief (Mindfulness Meditation, Volume One) by William M. Stanley (Kindle Edition)

- Personal Nutrition, Marie A. Boyle, Sara Long (Wadsworth Cengage Learning, Belmont, CA, 2010)

- Practical Aerobic Conditioning 2nd ed., Collins, D. Ray, Hodges Patrick B., John M. Kelly (Tichenor Publishing, Bloomington, Indiana, 1991)

- The Daniel Fast Diet: A Guide on How Christians can Lose Weight and Gain Spiritual Strength With the Daniel Fast.

- https://www.amazon.com/DANIEL-FAST-DIET-Christians-Spiritual-ebook/dp/B00SW3PUDE#navbar

# Endnotes

---

[1] http://gettinginshapeafter40.com/go/dieting-tips/

[2] http://www.christian-living-site.com/Temple-of-God.html

[3] http://gettinginshapeafter40.com/how-to-stay-motivated-to-lose-weight-2/

[4] http://www.affirmations.us/Weight-Loss-Affirmations.html

[5] http://www.lifepossibilities.com/

[6] Meditation Techniques: A Step-By-Step Guide on Using Meditation for Anxiety Relief (Mindfulness Meditation, Volume One) by William M. Stanley (Kindle Edition)http://www.amazon.com/gp/product/B00QB9897K

[7] https://www.humana.com/learning-center/health-and-wellbeing/mental-health/relax

[8] http://www.webmd.com/balance/stress-management/tc/aromatherapy-essential-oils-therapy-topic-overview

[9] http://www.amazon.com/Essential-Oils-proven-Aromatherapy-Beginners-ebook/dp/B00K5ZUKX2

[10] http://www.webmd.com/sleep-disorders/excessive-sleepiness-10/10-results-sleep-loss?page=3

[11] http://www.bodyandsoul.com.au/health/health+advice/10+benefits+of+a+good+nights+sleep,17681

[12] http://www.webmd.com/sleep-disorders/features/easy-snoring-remedies?page=3

[13] http://www.today.com/health/5-foods-may-make-you-feel-happier-now-even-better-t101030

[14] http://gettinginshapeafter40.com/good-protein-foods-to-eat-2/

[15] http://www.heart.org/HEARTORG/Healthy Living/HealthyEating/Nutrition/Fats-101_UCM_304494_Article.jsp#.V50nmRK GNVk

[16] http://www.livestrong.com/article/441906-

what-are-health-benefits-of-micronutrients/

[17] http://www.dummies.com/how-to/content/eating-clean-for-dummies-cheat-sheet.html

[18] https://www.humana.com/learning-center/health-and-wellbeing/diet-and-nutrition/foods-that-eat-up-the-pounds

[19] https://www.humana.com/learning-center/health-and-wellbeing/healthy-living/hangry

[20] http://blackdoctor.org/11660/how-to-eat-like-an-olympian/

[21]http://www.beliefnet.com/Faiths/Galleries/7-Bible-Verses-to-Motivate-You-to-Exercise.aspx?p=2#qbXQ0U6klBriGKpi.99

[22]https://www.adultfitnesstest.org/testInstructions/flexibility/sitAndReach.php

[23]http://www.cdc.gov/physicalactivity/basics/measuring/exertion.htm

[24] http://www.christian-living-site.com/Physical-Exercise.html

[25] https://www.verywell.com/how-much-exercise-do-you-really-need-1230940?utm_term=how+much+exercise+do+adults+need&utm_content=p1-main-2-title&utm_medium=sem-unp&utm_source=SEO&utm_campaign=&ad=SEO&an=SEO&am=&q=how+much+exercise+do+adults+need&o=&qsrc=&l=&askid=

[26] http://gettinginshapeafter40.com/exercising-tips-2/

[27] http://www.christian-living-site.com/Exercise-Routine.html

[28] http://www.mayoclinic.org/diseases-conditions/menopause/basics/definition/CON-20019726

[29] http://www.webmd.com/sex-relationships/low-testosterone-8/rm-quiz-truth-testosterone-html

[30] http://www.webmd.com/men/what-low-testosterone-can-mean-your-health

[31] http://www.ehow.com/how_2063616_rele

ase-endorphins.html

[32] http://www.cdc.gov/bloodpressure/facts.htm

[33] http://www.diabetes.org/diabetes-basics/symptoms/?loc=db-slabnav#sthash.8rwPcfS1.dpuf

[34] https://www.amazon.com/DANIEL-FAST-DIET-Christians-Spiritual-ebook/dp/B00SW3PUDE